My Fitness Entrepreneur: How to Become a Personal Trainer and Start a Personal Fitness Training Business

By Ahmed "Gino" Erguigue

Table of Contents

This book was brought to you by http://myfitnessentrepreneur.com

Introduction

Working as a personal trainer for the past 15 years has given me an extremely blessed life and I'm thankful every day that this is my profession. I love the fact that I get paid to positively impact the lives of my clients every single day. I put together this book to to help others achieve a career as rewarding as the one I've experienced. Hopefully this guide will help you find the same joy, satisfaction, and success that I have found in this dynamic profession.

This is my story and I hope you like it. It comes from my heart.

Gino

P.S. – If you have any questions or suggestions on how I can improve this guide, please let me know by contacting me through the contact page of my website! If you like this guide, please share it with anyone who may get some use out of it. That is the best kind of thank you I can get. The other best thank you is to leave a 4 or 5 star review for it on Amazon.

Note: Because recommended equipment and recommended supplements are constantly changing, that information can be found on these pages:

http://myfitnessentrepreneur.com/recommended-equipment/

http://myfitnessentrepreneur.com/recommended-supplements/

Section 1: Education and Certifications

Education and certification provide one of the most important aspects of building a career in the fitness industry: **credibility**. Expertise and continued self education is absolutely crucial in becoming successful (and it will facilitate every other aspect of operating a personal training business), so take it seriously!

Step 1. Meet current health and fitness professionals in your community.

If you want to be the best, you need to learn from the best. One of the best ways to start is to visit current fitness trainers working in your community.

Talk to them and learn from them. Tell them about your goals and the career you want to start. Anyone who is in this industry for the right reasons will be more than willing to share their experiences with you. Not only will you get lots of unique insights into the industry, you will be exposed to a wide range of philosophies within the health world.

Additionally, you will immediately develop a valuable network of contacts within your industry. It's a fantastic way to jump-start your business and show the world that you're serious about what you want to do. This is a huge advantage, regardless of whether you want to become a trainer working directly for a facility, or start your own training business.

Here are some places you can go to visit personal trainers:

⌖ Fitness Facilities Clubs

- Private Gyms
- Physical Therapy Clinics
- Sports Performance Centers (Strength and Conditioning)
- Hospital Wellness Centers
- Health and Wellness Centers

When visiting these places, see if you can set up a time to talk with one of the trainers to ask questions. You can ask about qualifications, personal trainer salary, the nature of fitness jobs in general, a typical day, etc. You can even ask to job shadow. Once you've done this in all of those places, you'll have a much more clear idea of what area you'd like to specialize in and then you can tailor your education accordingly.

Step 2. Get your education.

In order to become a fitness instructor, you need to become certified. Depending on your goals, an academic degree would also be useful in your career (but not necessary). Obviously those that opt to get a university degree in addition to their certifications will have an advantage in this industry, especially regarding employment options (or credibility if they are running their own business). Because getting a college degree is an expensive and lengthy process, you'll have to consider this option carefully. The first part of this process (talking to health and fitness professionals) should help you in deciding what is right for you.

A. University Degree

A lot of this stuff is obvious, so I won't get too in depth, but here is some advice if you do decide to get a degree in health education (or are considering it).

- Look into programs that specialize in Physical Education, Human Kinetics, Kinesiology, and other Human Movement Science programs.
- Talk to academic advisers, current students, and find out if mentors are offered (as well as post graduate job placement).
- Curriculums can be quite different in their course offering regarding whether they focus on theory or application, so try and find a program that has a nice balance of both.

Getting a college degree is a huge decision and not one to be taken lightly. In my personal opinion, it is absolutely worth it to do, and remember that you always have the option to get your degree while are you working as a trainer (going to college part time). I got my education and training from the **Athletic University of Rabat** (http://www.um5a.ac.ma/index.php/en/), Morocco (the National Academy of Sports Medicine) and it was a great decision for me.

Don't be discouraged because it takes a long time to get your degree. You can get a degree while you are working in the industry anyway. As Stephen Covey says, "It's not how fast you're going, but where you're headed that's most important."

B. Certifications

Getting certified is part of being a personal trainer and assists with your continued self education. But be sure to choose certifications wisely - there are a lot out there!

When choosing your certifications, you need to evaluate the following:

⅄ **Qualifications of the faculty of the certifying body**: Look at education levels, experience, and contribution to the field collectively. In other words, is it a legitimate certification? Where is it recognized? Be on the lookout for certifications that are meaningless.

⅄ **Curriculum**: Does it realistically help you work with the population you want to serve? Unless you are simply fascinated by the course topic, you want to focus on certifications that will help you with your clientele and your business. This means certifications that will give you credibility when you are trying to acquire new clients, as well as an education that will help serve your current clients.

Be sure to ask the local community / fitness centers for recognized programs in your city, province, or state. Realize that you will eventually need more than one certification.

You can never go wrong with getting certified through **NASM** (http://myfitnessentrepreneur.com/nasm), **ACE** (http://myfitnessentrepreneur.com/ace), **ISSA** (http://myfitnessentrepreneur.com/issa), or **NSCA** (http://myfitnessentrepreneur.com/nsca), since those are fairly well known and established personal training certifications. Once you have your basic level certification, you can investigate specialty certifications to further advance your skills (all are also available on those websites).

Once certified, it is only the beginning. To stay current, you need to continue to educate yourself. You can do this by reading regularly from the following:

⚞ **ACSM Health and Fitness Journal** (http://journals.lww.com/acsm-healthfitness/pages/default.aspx)

⚞ **IDEA Source** (http://www.ideafit.com/idea-health-fitness-source) and **IDEA Personal Trainer** (http://www.ideafit.com/idea-personal-trainer)

⚞ **NSCA Strength and Conditioning Journal and Journal of Strength and Conditioning Research** (http://www.nsca.com/publications/)

⚞ **Physician and Sportsmedicine** (https://www.physsportsmed.org/)

⚞ **Journal of Physiology** (http://onlinelibrary.wiley.com/journal/10.1111/%28ISSN%291469-7793)

⚞ **PTontheNET Publications** (http://www.ptonthenet.com/articles)

⚞ **Continuing Education Courses and Exams** (http://www.ptonthenet.com/cec-exams)

Your local college or university will also have many reputable journals where you can photocopy individual articles.

Every certification requires you to obtain a certain amount of contact hours taking courses to re-certify. This insures that their fitness professionals are continually upgrading and educating themselves. You can take many exciting courses in your local areas or by correspondence.

As mentioned above, taking a specialty certification further develops your skills. It also widens the population you can work with and this means greater income potential.

This book was brought to you by http://myfitnessentrepreneur.com

You have the opportunity to make an impact on someone's health in a positive way so be sure to take your education very seriously. Your clients (and your wallet!) will thank you!

C. CPR Certification

All personal trainer certifications require each member to become CPR certified. This is particularly important as a trainer because exercise causes various physiologic responses, that could result in unresponsiveness (this is rare but still possible). This could be a syncopal episode (passing out) or as extreme as an arrhythmia or cardiac arrest. CPR is indicated in a person who is not breathing or is apneic and has no pulse. Be sure to get your CPR certification and be ready to use that training if necessary.

Section 2: Training Philosphy

Now that you understand your educational obligations to be an effective trainer, it is time to start planning out your business. But before getting into the actual nuts and bolts of the business, it is first important to establish your training philosophy. Once you have these firmly established in your mind, it will make running every aspect of your business much easier.

Step 1. Set rules for working with your clients.

These are the rules you want to follow when working with your clients. While you are reading these rules you might think to yourself "all of these are really obvious." Well that may be true, but it is also true that these "obvious" rules are easy to break without even realizing it. I would suggest reading these regularly to remind yourself of how you want to interact with your clients. Print them out somewhere where you will read them everyday you go to work.

A. Don't train your clients like you train yourself.

This is one of the biggest mistakes I see in the personal training industry. A very minuscule percentage of your clients will think and act like you do, and therefore training them like you would train yourself simply won't work. When clients don't see the results they want or that they believed they'd get, they lose interest and drop out. If this develops into a pattern, your business won't build the clientele necessary to sustain it and you will fail. The easiest way to avoid this problem is to truly LISTEN to your client's wants and needs and set up a plan that will work for THEM. Just because you'd be able to follow it doesn't mean they will, so keep that in mind when doing your training.

B. Not all clients are the same.

As my wife (a physician) likes to say "treat the patient, not the disease." Each and every client has different goals, different body types, different metabolisms, and different lifestyles. Those cookie-cutter plans simply don't work for most people. If they did, personal trainers wouldn't even be necessary! Go the extra mile to make your clients feel like they are your only one and take a vested interest in their success. Remember that success for your clients means success for you and your business.

C. Don't mistake what the client wants / needs.

It's a huge mistake when a trainer doesn't find out what a client's goals are and confirm whether they're realistic and achievable. Clients with unrealistic goals are likely to drop out when they realize they aren't going to accomplish what they want. Make sure you have a clear understanding of what your client wants and let them know if their goal is realistic in the time frame desired. If it isn't, be honest with them and make sure they have a clear understanding of the results that can be achieved with your guidance.

D. Require discipline and commitment from your clients.

Certainly clients have more in their lives than their personal fitness goals, but when the trainer allows clients to miss sessions regularly or other forms of not following your training, those clients won't make any progress and will eventually drop out. Showing your client that you require discipline and commitment from them also reflects the amount of personal interest you have in their success. Your personal interest creates extra accountability and that can make all the difference.

Also, don't forget that a string of failures will ruin your reputation and jeopardize your business (whereas a string of success stories will do just the opposite).

Step 2. Set rules for yourself.

When you are running a personal training business, in essence the product you are selling is yourself. For that reason it is important that you set some philosophical rules for yourself as well. You are the foundation of your business and need to be optimal at all times.

Like I mentioned before, these may seem obvious, but that doesn't mean it's not easy to forget why you started in this business from time to time. I would also recommend reading these rules on a regular basis and printing them out somewhere where you will see them everyday you go to work.

A. Always be passionate.

My personal success has come from having a passion for helping others achieve their goals. I use my energy and enthusiasm for fitness to inspire others by leading by example. I am constantly reading about nutrition, athletic science, and fitness, which allows me to create unique and effective training programs that are personalized to each client. These programs are constantly changing to overcome plateaus and keep the client interested and motivated. This accompanied by great communication, an eye for detail, and exceptional teaching ability, along with a mastery of basic exercise techniques (i.e. progressions, regressions, and the principles of program design) are all qualities that turn a good trainer into a GREAT trainer. Most importantly you have to stay healthy because without your health, you cannot accomplish anything I have stated above. The people who truly see the power of health are those who don't have it, so be aware of it, appreciate it, and try to prolong it.

B. Invest in Self Education.

As I mentioned before, continued self education is the key to succeeding in this business and doing right by your clients. Knowledge builds confidence, so invest in your education, even after you've obtained your initial certifications. The organization that issues your certifications will let you know what you need to do to keep them current. Beyond that, you need to be reading and studying to stay up to date on fitness trends and news. Remember that studying current literature, attending classes, and going to conventions and conferences are all investments in your business, not expenses.

Section 3: Preparing for Business

At this point you should have a rough idea of what you sector of the industry you'd like to focus on through your conversations with fitness professionals, as well as figured out what kind of educational topics you'd like to specialize in. Knowing those things, along with your training philosophy rules for yourself and your clients, you're now ready to start setting up the nuts and bolts of your business, which will all be included on your website (you will be shown how to create a website in the next chapter).

Step 1. Create an availability schedule.

Decide in advance what days / hours per week you want to work, then create a schedule and stick to it. You may initially decide to work 12 hour days plus weekends, but that will get old fast, so I wouldn't recommend it. Organize a schedule that you know you will like and can commit to, and stick with that schedule. Remember that once you have offered availability to a client at specific times of the week and they accept, you are as committed as they are and can't back out (or if you do, it would look really bad).

Step 2. Decide what services you will be specializing in and what will be included in your plans.

This part is completely up to you and will depend largely on what you have chosen to study and what you are willing to offer. These can also be either included as part of your training sessions or something clients can purchase as an "add on" (such as nutrition / dieting plans to be given to them outside of the training sessions). I'll be showing you the payment plans I have set up in my training business later on.

Step 3. Decide how you will get paid.

If you are working as a personal trainer under a bigger company, they will most likely have some kind of payment system in place and you won't have to worry about this.

If you are running your own training business, you'll have to set up a method of receiving payments. When you are just starting out, an easy way to do this (outside of cash and checks) is using PayPal (http://myfitnessentrepreneur.com/paypal). You can accept payments in PayPal from other PayPal accounts, as well as credit and debit cards. You can put PayPal "pay now" buttons directly on your website (one time or recurring payments) and have people pay you through there. It's very easy to set up and use if you've never done it before.

Note: These payment buttons will go on hidden pages of your website since you don't want to announce your prices publicly (we'll cover why later on). An alternative option is to send invoices through emails via PayPal (also very easy to do).

Once your company has grown and you are ready for a more sophisticated payment and management system, you can invest in **Mind Body** (http://myfitnessentrepreneur.com/mindbody). This is software you can install directly on your website very easily and it will take care of online booking, payments, scheduling, and more (with a login area for all your clients). It is ideal for running your personal training business once you are more established.

Step 4. Create your client information database.

It is extremely important to build and maintain a database of current clients, former clients, and prospects who went through an initial consultation but didn't sign up (we will get to how to find new leads later on).

Be sure to keep it as up to date as possible and include as many details as possible! You want to remember absolutely everything about a client when you see them again, and this database will help you do that. When you first start off you can keep all this information on a simple Excel spreadsheet (endless columns for info). Once your company grows, I recommend moving on to using **Mind Body** (http://myfitnessentrepreneur.com/mindbody) to do this.

You'll be glad you've been doing this as more time starts to pass. Don't think that your memory will serve you and you'll remember everything about every single prospect or client you've met (you won't). With this database you can be prepared before you see this person again. "In the previous training package you lost 16 lbs over 24 sessions!" "Last time I saw you you said you couldn't sign up because you were too busy with school, but now we're in summer!" Things like that is what this database is very useful for. Don't be lazy and include all the details you can!

Section 4: Advertising Your Services

You now have everything ready to go except for one thing: the clients! The goal here is to not only generate new leads for your business in the most effective way possible, but to have these leads already sold on your services before they even meet you! This is done by establishing credibility and the best way to do that is to create a website that showcases your expertise and your services.

Step 1. Create a website for your business (I'll show you how to do this in less than two hours total).

A professional website will give you unmatched credibility that you are serious about your business and what you do. By the time a potential client meets you, they should already be convinced of your effectiveness as a trainer without you having to say anything at all. This is a huge advantage for closing leads and will have a large impact on your business.

Once you have your website up (we'll go over how to do that in a minute - it's very easy), the basic method for advertising is really simple: announce your services in all the ways that you can think of (business cards, fliers, posters, etc.) and put your website address on every single one of them.

The website address being on all your advertisements is crucial. See, nobody wants to contact someone they don't know anything about, which is why all those advertising methods are useless if you only have your contact information on there. A website they can check out first is much more inviting and will make it much more likely that a potential client will reach out to you.

If you want to make all of this really happen, build a website for your business. With a website you will instantly become legitimate in everyone's eyes. Not only that, once you have your website up, this will all become an official business instead of some idea you are kicking around in your head. Building a website for your business will force you to organize your business and put it down somewhere public where everyone can see it.

When creating your website, be sure to include your education, certifications, philosophy, testimonials (I will go over testimonials later), services, and any other details that you'd like. This is also a great place to include recommended supplements, equipment, and basic dieting information (once you're a trainer you'll be asked about these things all the time, and now you'll have a website to refer people to). I would suggest building your website right away.

Note: When building your website, do NOT include specifics about the plans you are offering or prices at all. Keep that part vague! I will explain why later. :D

Building a website is actually a very simple and inexpensive process and I'm going to have my friend Mike Omar of the **Make Money from Home LIONS CLUB** (http://makemoneyfromhomelionsclub.com/) take over this chapter and provide the instructions on how to build one.

Mike Omar:

I'd like to add to what Gino said and introduce the idea of creating a blog for your business as well (the blog can be on a tab of your training website or on a separate website altogether). Blogging is something you can start to do even if you're not ready to launch your training business yet.

This book was brought to you by http://myfitnessentrepreneur.com

Blogging is a valuable, simple, and inexpensive tool that can be used for exploring topics, sharing ideas, connecting with others, and building businesses. It can lead to unexpected personal and business opportunities, as well as clarity of mind and purpose. Blogging, combined with the power of social media, is one of the most powerful tools for massive exposure that exists today. I highly recommend starting a blog, as part of, or in addition to, your personal training website.

Whether you decide to start a website, a blog, or both, the process is exactly the same.

Today I'm going to show you how to make a website (or blog) on its own domain, without coding, using WordPress (it's a surprisingly simple process). These are professional websites with any look that you want (and can incorporate anything that you want, including social media buttons, "buy now" buttons, mailing list forms, Google maps, etc.).

Note: When I say we will be creating a website using WordPress, I don't mean creating one through the WordPress website. Websites created through there are severely limited in what you can do with them and offer very little flexibility overall. The method I teach enables you to create truly professional websites by installing the WordPress software and you won't be limited in any way.

Not only is WordPress very easy to use, it is 100% free and makes your website completely customizable. Over 15% of websites online have been created with WordPress; if you can use Microsoft Word, you can make a website using WordPress (the website
Make Money from Home LIONS

CLUB (http://makemoneyfromhomelionsclub.com/) was made using WordPress…and I don't even know any code!).

Set aside one hour and make your first website TODAY!

What will be the total cost of your website? About $15 / year for the domain and $10 / month for hosting (the hosting can be used for as many domains as you want, so the price never goes up).

You can watch the entire process of me creating a basic blog on its own domain on the YouTube video on this website all in less than 15 minutes: **Mike Omar Photography** (http://mikeomarphotography.com/).

This is the first of four video lessons where I will show you the entire completion of the website **Mike Omar Photography** (http://mikeomarphotography.com/) ALL IN UNDER ONE HOUR TOTAL! Follow along in the video lessons and you'll see just how easy it is to build a website. :D

To watch the remaining three video lessons to complete your website, click here: **How to Make a Website or Blog using WordPress without Coding on your own Domain** (http://makemoneyfromhomelionsclub.com/udemyenglish1). Just register with Udemy and you'll have access to all the video lessons (it's completely free). If you are interested in watching additional free video lessons on home entrepreneurship and how to build an online business, visit the **Make Money from Home LIONS CLUB** (http://makemoneyfromhomelionsclub.com/).

"Like" or share my Udemy course if you liked it, and feel free to message me directly if you have any questions (contact information can be found on my website).

This book was brought to you by http://myfitnessentrepreneur.com

If you are interested in blogging about fitness / nutrition / health / etc., you may be interested in my book: **How to Start a Blog that People Will Read** (http://makemoneyfromhomelionsclub.com/ebookblog). The book focuses on how to make money blogging about a topic you love. This includes how to strategically pick your blog topics and write your blog posts (based on keyword research), as well as how to best monetize your blog, promotional strategies that will drive traffic to your blog, and how to create a growing and loyal readership.

Section 5: The Power of Testimonials

I'm sure that you've heard that word of mouth is the best form of advertisement. This is true, and there is nothing more powerful then having your current clients sell to your prospects in the form of success stories. Testimonials are hands-down the most effective way to demonstrate your effectiveness as a personal trainer.

Step 1. Get testimonials and list them on your website.

I realize this is a bit of a catch-22 at first since you won't have any clients to be your testimonials, but as soon as you get your first string of success stories, ask them if they would like to a be a testimonial for you. A client happy with the results will almost always say yes. Ask them to write a testimonial for you, as well as a few before and after pictures, and put those up on your website. There is nothing more powerful than these images; they will drive the value of your training program.

Just to show you how effective they are, I am going to put some of my own testimonials right here below. I can guarantee these testimonials will be what give me the most credibility out of everything you have seen so far.

Testimonial 1:

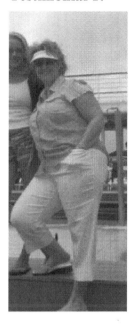

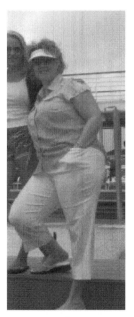

Before

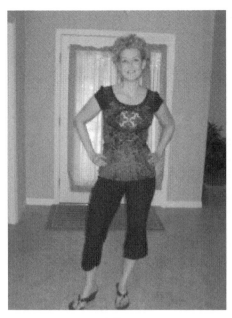

After

"There is no greater feeling than accomplishing what seems to feel impossible. For me, the decision came down to if I really wanted to be unhappy living the rest of my life the way I was when I was overweight. And for me, it just wasn't an option anymore. It simply becomes a choice. I am not saying it was easy. It absolutely wasn't. It took hard work and determination and the most important thing was diet and preparation. I can tell you there is no greater feeling than toughing it out and conquering one of the greatest challenges in front of you. And as you see progress happen every week, it drives you to push even harder. Gino was a great inspiration teaching me new things I never would have tried before to break through my plateaus and pushing me on those days I felt discouraged. He was there to help me on this journey every step of the way. And on those days that you fell miserable and discouraged, he was always there to make you laugh and help fix your spirit so you wouldn't give up. Never give up hope and never give up trying because IT WILL CHANGE YOUR LIFE!!!!" - Christine Grodzki

Testimonial 2:

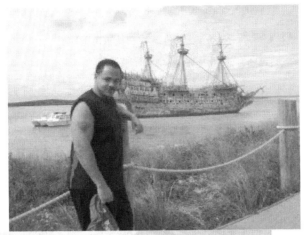

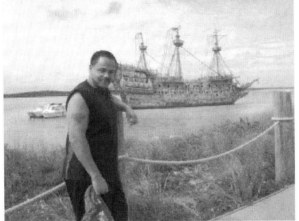

Before

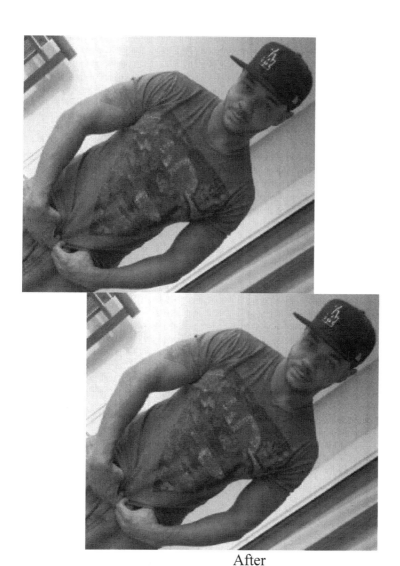

After

"I just want to take a few minutes to show my appreciation my personal trainer Gino. When I first started working out with him I was overweight and completely out of shape. I knew I needed a change in my life. Gino challenged me to that change and told me I will get out of it what I put into it. The training was not easy but I stuck with it and after a few weeks I started seeing great results. As my motivation increased my confidence did as well. After working with Gino I lost over 30 pounds and now I don't get discouraged looking in the mirror anymore. Gino not only changed my body but he changed my life. THANK YOU GINO!!" - Sha-Ron Dean

Testimonial 3:

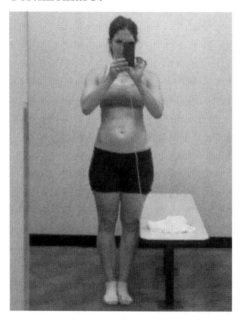

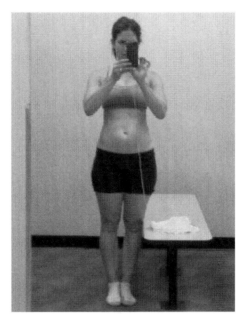

Before

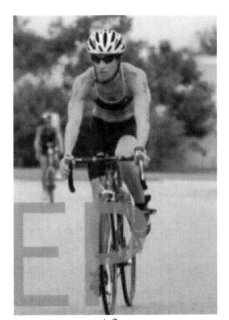

After

This book was brought to you by http://myfitnessentrepreneur.com

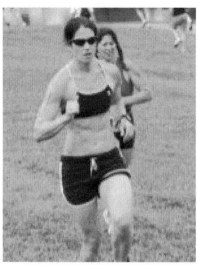
After

"I want to encourage anyone considering the investment of hiring a personal trainer to take on the great challenge of the work Gino will put you through. I have been an "athlete" most of my life and in team sports throughout high school, college and then later while looking for the camaraderie of sport started competing in sprint distance tri's. Many times I've been asked "why do you use a personal trainer if you know what to do?". There's nothing like having a great coach to push you through and out of your comfort zone to gain your greatest potential. Gino has given me the tools to constantly keep me engaged, challenged and motivated to get better even when life's challenges get in the way, as they do for all of us. As a mother of three (9 yrs, 8yrs & 10months old), wife and business owner things are constantly shifting and time becomes less and less available. What I can say with absolute confidence is that a training day with Gino will help keep me focused on "me" to push through and be better at the other areas of my life that are so incredibly important! Gino is honest, incredibly knowledgeable and professional. I am certain that should you take on the challenge to train with Gino it will be the best investment in YOU!" - Daniela Montiel

Testimonial 4:

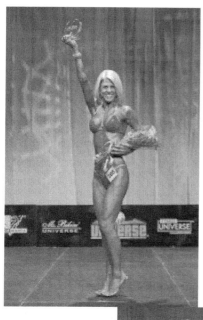

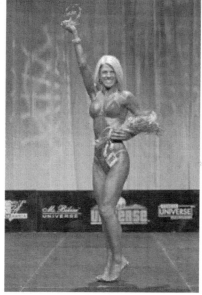

After

"I have been training for the past eleven weeks with Gino Erguigue. I am preparing to compete in Ms. Bikini at Fitness Universe in Miami in June. I approached Gino three months ago,

This book was brought to you by http://myfitnessentrepreneur.com

handed him a picture of a Fitness Model with six pack abs , and said " Can you give me abs like hers?" Gino's knowledge and ability to use so many different cardio and weight workouts, along with putting me on an eat-clean diet, has transformed not only my abs, but my entire body. GIno motivated me to push myself harder then I thought was physically possible. I am four weeks out from my competition and I am amazed with how my body has changed in just eleven weeks of training with Gino. I am looking forward to seeing the end result in four more weeks. I have learned that with motivation, dedication, determination, an eat-clean diet, and a knowledgable trainer, anything is attainable." - Torraine Sarro

The longer you are in business, the more testimonials you will collect, so keep collecting them as you continue to grow. There is no limit. :D

Section 6: Closing Your Leads and Sample Pricing Plans

Everything you have done has brought you to this point: it's time to meet your potential client for the first time and close the deal. If they've found you through your advertising and have seen your website (and your testimonials), you already have a lot of credibility and this should go much more smoothly. If they know nothing about you, it will be tougher (but obviously still doable).

Step 1. Prepare for the initial meeting.

Like I've said before, most of the sale should be done before your prospect actually meets you, and when they finally do, everything about you should reflect total professionalism. Selling personal training is about confidence, so never miss an opportunity by always being prepared.

A. Make a strong first impression.

Be warm and welcoming with a smile, a firm handshake, and good eye contact. Maintain a quite confidence, but make sure to not be cocky! A cocky attitude can kill your sale very quickly because it can turn people off. During this initial small talk, you want to be warm and friendly (making the prospect feel comfortable is key) while establishing an air of professionalism.

Don't ever forget that all prospects are created equal. The biggest mistake personal trainers make is prejudging prospects. Don't be someone who clearly treats different people differently (as so many trainers do), based on things like how much money you think someone has or how much you may want to work with someone.

This book was brought to you by http://myfitnessentrepreneur.com

Not only is doing that in poor taste, it will negatively impact your business overall.

It doesn't matter if a potential client is old or young, attractive or ugly, poor or rich, male or female, skinny or overweight, etc.; they all need to be treated with respect. Sure, all trainers would love to train world class athletes that love a challenge and will do whatever you say, but that isn't the reality. Everyone who you meet deserves to be treated like a person that you would love to work with (just like everyone you do train deserves the best service you can give them).

Remember that a gym is as much a place to socialize as it is to workout, and people talk. If you develop a reputation for acting this way (playing favorites, etc.), it will hurt your business.

Step 2. Learn how to direct a typical conversation with a new potential client.

Now that you've done some small talk, it is time to move on to the selling part of the conversation. There is already a ton of material that exists about how to be a good salesperson, so we're just going to focus on the things you need to think about in this profession. Let's go over how a typical conversation goes in one of these first-time meetings and how you need to think and act to close the sale.

A. How to direct the beginning of the conversation.

A potential client usually has these questions in mind and will sometimes start with one of these questions right away:

⋏ How much does this cost?

- How often do I need to see you?
- What do I need to do to lose x .lbs?
- How quickly will I see results?
- I just want a program for you to design but for me to do on my own. Can you do that?

Don't answer these question. Doing so will decrease your chances of making the sale or disable you from selling a bigger package than the client initially thought that they wanted.

Remember: the client has taken time out of their busy day to come see you. You are in the position of power and should be controlling the conversation, not them. Immediately after the small talk is over, ask him or her "what is it you want to achieve?" and let them talk. It shifts control of the conversation and puts you in the drivers seat. Listen to what the person tells you and take careful notes. Have a pad of paper and pen ready; active note-taking is important in making the clients know that you care. When the client stops talking, just wait. In silence, they will usually start talking again. All of the information they are giving you is ammunition for when you go to make the sale.

If a client keeps quiet after they've been talking, ask if there is a specific reason why he or she is coming to you. Listen carefully to their **emotional** reason for sitting in the chair across from you. Why do they want to lose x .lbs? Always remember that emotion is what drives action. It's important during this initial part of the meeting to be quiet and let the client speak. Often all I do is ask questions.

Here are some of the questions I usually ask during these initial meetings (depending on the direction the conversation goes):

⅄ What is it you want to achieve?

⅄ What is the specific reason you came to see me? **Note:** If they say something like "to find out how much this costs" you say "well what are your goals?"

⅄ What are you goals?

⅄ Have you been a member of a gym before?

⅄ Have you had a trainer before?

⅄ Why did you quit or not achieve your goal?

⅄ If you could overcome these challenges, what would your new physique look like?

⅄ If you accomplish your goals, what would this mean for your life?

⅄ If you don't accomplish your goals, what difficulties will you continue to face or might you face in the future?

⅄ What are you expectations of me?

Notice that all the questions are open-ended questions (not "yes" or "no" questions). These keep the potential client talking.

Now that you have an idea of what they want, move to more technical questions:

⅄ How much time are you willing to dedicate to these goals?

⅄ What is your schedule like?

⅄ How many times per week are you currently working out?

⅄ How many times per week would you like to workout?

⅄ What are some of your likes and dislikes when training?

⅄ Do you have any injuries or complications I should be aware of?

Notice how much information we have and how specific we have gotten without ever talking about price. This entire time you want to be relaxed, listening with interest (writing things down of course!), and showing empathy. Only respond when necessary and always maintain self control (don't seem as if you are waiting to start selling). Get all the information you can before you even start to think about selling.

Creating a foundation of trust and respect is not only crucial for getting the sale, it will also establish a baseline for the rest of your relationship (in other words, it will also make the training of the client easier later on). A client that trusts and respects you will listen more, and therefore get better results, and therefore stay longer as a client, as well as increase your reputation as a good trainer. Remember that this is a team effort from here on out!

Once you know what the client hopes to achieve, as well as their preferences and how much time they can commit, give them an idea of your plan on a piece of paper in front of the client explaining it step by step. Explain why your plan is specifically suited to get them their results. Be brief to start. Let the client lead you in terms of how much detail you provide. I have found that some clients were more interested in the physiology behind adaptation. Some don't care and just want results. Let your client lead how you describe your program. Remember that you're an expert when sitting in a sales meeting. Inform the client of what they can expect by training with you and make sure the client has a good idea of what you are offering. Let them know what the game plan is.

This is also a good time to show them photos of your testimonials from your website to really drive the point home on the effectiveness of your programs (if a computer with Internet isn't available, make sure you have your testimonials printed out for the meeting!).

Before bringing up price you should book the person into your schedule according to the plan you have outlined, having clients commit to training times and dates. They will commit to whatever you propose so always suggest a higher number of training sessions per week to start off.

After all this, it is finally time to reveal the price of your program.

B. Discussing price and sample pricing structure.

I suggest you have a professional sales sheet with 4 different pricing plans for each length of time offered.

Depending on your qualifications, experience, location, clientele base, etc., you can modify these prices as you see fit, but this is the pricing structure of the plans I offer:

30 minutes per session pricing:

8 sessions ----- $75 each

16 sessions ----- $70 each

24 sessions ----- $65 each

48 sessions ----- $60 each

1 hour per session pricing:

8 sessions ----- $115 each

16 sessions ----- $110 each

24 sessions ----- $105 each

48 sessions ----- $100 each

Be gentle and break down what they are paying for! Emphasize that a half hour or hour with you is much more effective than a half hour or hour by themselves. Also remember that the program you are offering is worth every penny and be firm about it. The cheapest trainer in the world is too expensive if the client isn't sold on your value. You are the product, so believe in its value and learn to communicate it to the client.

When you present the options, you will find most people will buy one of the middle packages. There are also some people that will always buy the most expensive thing you present, which is why we have a 48 session package in there (just in case).

C. Overcoming objections.

Once you've finished describing the payment plans, say something like "what do you think about the overall game plan?" and listen to what they have to say.

These are typically the biggest objections:

> ⚔ **Money**: This is the biggest one. This is why you need to sell value during the entire meeting and only mention the price at the end. If you tell them the price at the beginning and they don't like it, you may lose them right off the bat and nothing else you say will matter. Your rebuttals at this point could be things like "are you willing to sacrifice certain pleasures to reach your goals?" or "this is one of the most important investments of your life."

⅄ **Lack of time**: This shouldn't be an issue because you already know their time constraints and made a plan according to their needs. Even so, it can still come up as an objection. This can be overcome by continuing to modify your plan within their schedule. Remind them that everyone has at least a spare 2-3 hours per week (and they wouldn't be taking the meeting with you if they didn't).

⅄ **Injury**: Make sure you understand the injury fully and add that information into the database for later followup.

⅄ **Age**: Some clients are convinced that they are either too old or too young (or too "whatever") for a training program. This is simply untrue: absolutely anyone can benefit from conditioning the body and will feel better as a result.

⅄ **Already in shape**: Some clients will already be in great shape naturally and wonder why they might need your services. You might remind them to watch out for complacency and tell them that staying in shape is significantly easier than to fall out of shape and then come back to their original state later on.

⅄ **"Know it all" attitude**: Many clients believe that they don't need a trainer because they know what they're doing and they simply ask for a workout plan. Clients with this "know it all" attitude usually need a softer approach. Emphasize your expertise; it is unlikely that someone will know more than you do, and in the unlikely event that they do, they will see the value in having a trainer anyway. Having a trainer will always be more effective than training alone.

⚔ **"I need to think about it"**: Try and dig deeper and find out the real reason they are hesitant. If you can't get that information, make sure the client understands your value and payment plans before they leave.

One final technique: If a client isn't sure and is taking too much time to make a decision (and they clearly aren't going to say "yes" at this point), as a final resort you can say something like "I can see you don't want this badly enough and I don't want both of us to waste our time." Because they see that you are about to take away their opportunity to train with you, they suddenly want it. I've had several clients sign up on the spot using this tactic.

Remember that successful health and fitness professionals keep in consistent contact. They understand that a "no" today is not a "no" indefinitely. That client may come back at a later date or may refer someone else (even if they themselves said no). This is why it is important to always stay professional regardless of the outcome of these meetings.

D. What to do when a client says "yes".

When a prospect says ' yes ' you have to go through the following steps:

1. Collect payment (can be cash, check, through **PayPal** (http://myfitnessentrepreneur.com/paypal) or through **Mind Body** (http://myfitnessentrepreneur.com/mindbody)).

2. Schedule the client's first appointment (and make sure it is within 48 hours of that meeting if possible).

3. Congratulate your client on taking the first step toward their goal.

4. Send your client a thank you card within 24 hours.

Section 7: Maintenance and Growth

At this point you have passed the initial phase of launching your business and you are now in maintenance / growth mode. This final segment of your business is certainly the easiest: your advertising methods are already in place, you have existing clients referring new ones, and your reputation is already established and continues to grow stronger. All you have to do is keep your current clients happy.

Step 1: Steadily build your client base.

This is a process that certainly does not happen overnight. This takes years of good training and referrals from happy customers. It involves making yourself known in your local community as well as the internet and various forms of social media. Many organizations now offer a trainer referral system. Additionally, associations such as **ACE** (http://myfitnessentrepreneur.com/ace) and **NSCA** (http://myfitnessentrepreneur.com/nsca) are actively advertising their own trainers to the public. For as little as $25.00 a year, you can place your bio and website on these websites. These very same organizations also offer discussion boards where the public can come to find information and access personal trainers. Post on these websites offering helpful information and a link back to your website. It's a very effective method of gaining credibility while recruiting potential clients at the same time.

Step 2. Don't ever lose focus of your clients.

Here are just a few final things to keep in mind when working with your current clients:

This book was brought to you by http://myfitnessentrepreneur.com

⅄ Keep treating your current clients like gold, build long lasting relationships with them, and never take them for granted; renewing contacts with existing clients is easier than finding new ones and this will keep your business more steady in the long run.

⅄ Change up the routines of your existing clients to keep things interesting and challenging. Be sure to keep measuring their progress.

⅄ Always maintain open and honest communication. This will keep clients from unexpectedly dropping out of your services (and will give you a chance to keep this from happening if you already know that they are thinking about it).

⅄ Don't forget why your clients signed up with you in the first place and keep up your commitment to them!

⅄ Remind your clients that the best thank you they can give is a referral. I usually thank clients with a free session for every referral they give me to make it known that I appreciate what they did.

Health and Fitness Evaluation Form

Gino Erguigue, NASM-CPT, NSCA-CSCS

The purpose of this evaluation is to have a clear understanding of your present *lifestyle*, discuss your *fitness goals*, as well as encourage an understanding of their crucial relationship to one another. This will help me narrow down a more specialized health and fitness plan that suits your individual needs.

Name:_____

Date:_____

Address:_____

_____

Phone:_____

Alt#:_____

Email:_____

Age:_____

1) What are your top 3 fitness goals?

2) In what physical activities are you currently involved and how often do you participate?

3) What is your occupation? (specify)

This book was brought to you by http://myfitnessentrepreneur.com
Page 47

4) Have you had any surgery the last year? (specify)

5) Have you had a history of any of the following: (circle all that apply)

Asthma Y N

High Blood Pressure Y N

Heart Disease Y N

Stroke Y N

Diabetes Y N

Hernia Y N

6) Hours of sleep per night:

7) Have you ever experienced dizziness/fainting?

8) Please list your current medications and the condition (if any):

9) Do you have any bone or joint problems (i.e. Arthritis)? (Specify)

10) Have you ever had a major injury to any joint or part of your musculoskeletal system? Please specify.

11) Are you currently receiving physical therapy? If yes, for what condition?

12) What known physical limitations do you have (personally or doctor prescribed)?

13) Please circle or check off the activities below that are of any interest to you?

Weight reduction
Flexibility

Muscle building   Cycling

Muscle toning   Yoga/ Pilates

Cardiovascular training   Sport-specific training

Marathon/triathlon training   Nutrition

Boxing/combat aerobics   Bodybuilding/Figure/Fitness competition

Weight loss/ Body fat reduction   Sprinting and agility training

*All the information I have disclosed in this form in true to the best of my knowledge and I will notify my personal trainer immediately if any changes arise.

Client Signature:_____

Date:_____/_____/_____

Personal Trainer:

_____ Date:_____/_____/_____

PROGRESS TRACKER

Date:__/__/__

Height:____Weight:_____BP:___/___BMI:____BF%:____C/A/H/
T/A:__/__/__/__/__

Measurements: Date:_____ Date:_____ Date:_____

Weight: _____ _____ _____

BMI: _____ _____ _____

BF%: _____ _____ _____

Chest: _____ _____ _____

Abs: _____ _____ _____

Hips: _____ _____ _____

Upper thigh: _____ _____ _____

Upper arm: _____ _____ _____

Personal Trainer Contract

I, Ahmed (Gino) Erguigue, have received payment in full from client, _____, in the amount of $_____ via a personal check / cash (circle one) on today's date_____. This sum entitles client to _____, one-hour personal training sessions at a rate of $_____/session, on/at a mutually convenient date and time. If a cancellation is necessary, a text/phone call 24-hr prior to the scheduled session is required to avoid payment for that individual session. The training sessions must be completed within ____ days of the above contract date. I agree that this sale is final and there are absolutely no refunds after three business days.

Client Signature:_____

Date:_____

Personal Trainer Signature:_____

Date:_____

Ahmed (Gino) Erguigue, NASM-CPT, NSCA-CSCS

xxx-xxx-xxxx

email@gmail.com

Session Completion Signature Sheet

Gino Erguigue, NASM-CPT, NSCA-CSCS

Client:_____ Phone:
_____

Package Under Contract:_____ Date package
purchased:___/___/___

Date	Time	Client Signature	Session	Trainer Initials

Case Study: How to Open a Gym or Fitness Training Facility (the blunt truth).

If you are interested in opening your own gym or fitness training facility, my experience might be able to help. I don't have a background in business or anything like that, but I did help my friend successfully open a gym in Orlando several years ago. I am happy to tell you about how that went here, and hopefully this will help you out if you are trying to accomplish something similar.

I'm going to assume you already have a background in fitness. If you don't, stop reading this right now because it is not a smart idea for you to try and open a gym (or any type of fitness training club) if you don't have a background in fitness and haven't worked at some type of fitness center for at least a few years. That experience will help you tremendously in terms of how to operate and grow a successful training facility (much more than can be learned through reading about it anywhere). It will be the key to making sure you are making good decisions regarding location, prices for services, employee compensation, creating policies, etc. If this is something you really want to do, I highly recommend getting a job at a gym first and work a few different positions.

The rest of the information you'll need in order to do this successfully can be learned through general small-business guides (to learn about different legal business classifications, bookkeeping, taxes, banking, paperwork, etc.).

So what's left? This is the blunt truth about what it takes to launch this business, how to be realistic about your expectations the first few years of operation, and actual earnings you might expect.

This book was brought to you by http://myfitnessentrepreneur.com

1. Estimate your expenses and revenue.

Based on your vision of the type of training center you'd like to open, find an appropriate location and figure out your total expenses for your first year. This includes rent (or down payment plus mortgage), electricity / utilities, equipment (could be purchased or leased), insurance (about $200 / month to cover members), and any other expenses you can think of. Now take that number of total first year expenses and double it.

Then figure out your expected revenue for each month for the first year (based on expected new customers, recurring membership dues, expected training contracts, etc.). Once you have those numbers, take your entire expected revenue for the first year and cut it in half. Now subtract your first year expenses from your first year revenues (the number should be negative).

This number is the very least amount of capital you should raise to start this venture. Now project how your second year and third years will go using the same rules (double your monthly expenses and halve your monthly expected revenue). If you can get break through to the point where your business is making a livable profit monthly (after you've included your payment schedule to your investors), you have a chance to make this work (I don't mean to sound bleak, but this is realistic).

Here was his gym's approximate breakdown for revenue:

⋏ Membership dues - 70%

⋏ Personal training lot rent (from 2 sub-contracted trainers) - 25%

⋏ Merchandise and supplement sales - 5%

2. Raise capital.

Now that you know how much you need to start your business, it is time to figure out how you're going to obtain the necessary capital. Unless you're independently wealthy, you will most likely need investors. Start inquiring with clients, friends, family, etc., to see if anyone has any interest. Find out what they're interested in for a return on their investment (could be equity or a return on their loan).

It might be possible to find other business owners that need an additional expense off their bottom line (for tax purposes), so investing in your business will serve their purpose. If possible, find someone like that. Another option is to try and get a loan from a bank.

For any of these options, you're going to have to write a business plan (it's very unlikely that any potential investor is going to give up their money if you don't have a detailed plan). Using a business plan program to write your business is an easy way to get this done (my friend used **Business Plan Pro** (http://myfitnessentrepreneur.com/businessplanpro)). That program is very easy to use and will provide information that you wouldn't have taken into account otherwise.

Also, find a way to invest your own money (my friend used a home equity line, which is basically a second mortgage). It's also unlikely that any investor is going to give up their money if they don't see that you're willing to take a risk too.

3. Be prepared to work.

Like personal training, operating a gym is not as easy as it might seem from a distance. You have to be persistent and love what you do. If not, it will never work. Be ready to jeopardize your relationships and have most people have zero appreciation for just how much work it is to keep the doors open. Not to mention the extra weight on your shoulders that comes with owning your own business; this is something you can't really appreciate until you've done it yourself.

That being said, also be excited to change lives positively, build relationships that will last a lifetime, and never have to work for someone else ever again (another thing that you can't really appreciate until you've done it yourself).

In terms of money made, I know for a fact that it took my friend a few years to start profiting in the six figures (and the money did continue to grow). But for the first three years, be prepared to work constantly for very little compensation and remember that the possibility of failing is real.

Take the time to put thought into what you're doing before you make your final decision. Good luck!

Top 16 Mistakes Personal Trainers Make

1. Not doing the initial assessment with new clients. This is the worst thing you can do to your client. You have to do this in order to properly figure out what goals are attainable for your client as well as design a fitness plan that will work best specifically for them.

2. Not being confident or being scared of sales. Lack of communication or poor body language can affect your sales drastically. The best trainers I've ever seen followed one simple trick which led to their success: they made sure to introduce themselves to at least one stranger every day. They did this on the bus, in the coffee shop, on the street, or in the gym. If you can strike up a conversation with a stranger, then you can definitely sell the one product in the world you truly believe in: YOURSELF.

3. Recommending supplements just to get a commission. Your reputation is your biggest asset. It takes years to build and only one mistake to break. Promoting supplements may seem like a good way to make passive income, but I can't stress enough how careful you need to be when going down this route. There are a number of different companies that offer commission structures for trainers that promote and sell their supplements to their clients. The reality is that most clients won't benefit from supplements; generally speaking, eating whole foods and getting consistent work outs are the most important factors. Only recommend supplements that you truly believe in and that will really benefit that client, regardless of whether you get a commission or not.

4. Taking clients from other trainers. This is a touchy subject. If you do a great job (and if you're reading this, I assume you do or

This book was brought to you by http://myfitnessentrepreneur.com

will), then clients will ask to train with you if they're unsatisfied with their trainer. In situations like this, have the client let that trainer know of their decision, and then talk to that trainer yourself and let them know the decision was made entirely by the client. You want to have a good relationship with other trainers (you can even offer to help in any way that you can, just be careful not to hurt their pride).

If you are working at a gym and this happens, you can approach your manager and have them make the switch. This disconnects you from the situation.

Regardless of how the switch is finally made, **never** speak poorly of other trainers.

5. Not smiling, making eye contact, or being friendly. You're in the relationship business and you need to be approachable (not intimidating!). When a client walks in the door, a big smile says "I'm happy to see you" and engages them right away. You have the best job in the world, so show it!

6. Being lazy when designing training programs for your clients. Your job is to give your clients a workout specific to them. Don't get lazy; really focus on making the best program you possibly can (and continuously update it to keep challenging your client). You have to care and focus on your client's goals and that will show through your passion for your job.

7. Not gathering testimonials. Ask new clients if they would be willing to take some photos before they start training with you, and then later on as they continue to make progress. Once you have some good before and after photos, ask the client if they would be willing to write a testimonial for you (if they've had success, they will almost certainly say yes). Then put all that information on your website.

If your client gives you a great compliment, ask them to write it down and also put it on your website. You can never have too many testimonials.

From day one you should be gathering as many testimonials as possible. They are one of the most powerful ways of demonstrating that you can train effectively. Prospective clients see these and automatically think that they can accomplish what all of your other clients have accomplished if they sign up for your services.

8. Not caring about the profession. Personal training is a physically exhausting profession and will wear you down if you're motivation is purely financial. You have to love your clients, love everything related to fitness, and love bettering yourself. Personal training isn't a profession that you can simply coast through; it's a hustle. You must always be on at all hours of the day (especially when you are with your clients). It's impossible to do well unless you love the job.

9. Not keeping track of your client's progress. Walk into any gym and an easy way to tell whether a trainer is serious about their job is whether they're carrying a clipboard. It doesn't matter what method you use to monitor the workouts, but every set, rep and weight should be tracked. Do this both to improve your clients' results and also to protect yourself legally.

10. Working too much and burning out. Sure, it sounds like a good idea to work as much as possible. That way you make the most money, right? Wrong. Schedule your clients in bunches. Figure out the times you want to work during the week and only

This book was brought to you by http://myfitnessentrepreneur.com

put clients within those slots. If you feel like you need a break and aren't excited to go into the gym anymore, then take a long weekend. Disconnect and get some rest. Exhaustion creeps up on trainers. The money lost while taking a short rest will come back ten-fold if you do a great job instead of a mediocre one.

11. Not having a website and business cards. If you don't have these yet, stop reading right now and get this taken care of! Create your website and then get business cards with your name, contact info, and web address on there. It doesn't have to be anything fancy and both are easy / cheap to do. Every single one of your clients should have your business card and you should always have at least 10 in your wallet at all times.

12. Not working with other trainers. Textbooks and workshops are always great for improving your craft, but the best resource for learning is other trainers. Arranging a one hour block of time once a week with 1-2 other trainers for a communal workout is a great way to pick up new tricks and practice old ones. Pick a topic for the day and leave the workout open-ended. Theory has its time and place, but nothing can replace practical experience from people already successfully using it.

13. Using the same program for every client. It's ok to have a template. In fact, I'll go so far as to recommend you use the same template for every type of client you deal with. Why not? If you find a type of programming that works for fat loss clients stick to it. The same goes for hypertrophy clients and so on.

However, the best trainers are those who are able to adapt the same protocol for the individual. Changing up seemingly small details (such as the grip on an exercise or things like that) can make a big difference for clients with particular needs. Figure out what works and stick to it, but make sure to individualize it whenever it's needed.

14. Talking too much about yourself. I'll admit that I fall in this trap myself. The time spent in sessions belongs to your client, so try your best to keep the focus on them. If they ask a question about you, don't skimp on the details, but be sure to follow up with a question about them.

15. Not correcting technique / expecting perfect form. "Good" is not great and "good" won't suffice. Your clients should be great. Always be correcting and improving their technique, and never be satisfied. Constant little cues are the best way to make technique a habit for your clients and have them learn a new skill perfectly.

16. Not introducing yourself to every member of the gym. The most successful trainers in a gym setting are the most popular ones. They're the people who are on the floor saying hi to the members by name and introducing themselves to new members. The more approachable you make yourself in the gym, the more likely people will ask you about training.

I've never asked for a member off of the floor to train with me. Instead, I've introduced myself and helped them with whatever they had a question with. I also send them info afterwards if I have an article with more info. The member may not immediately ask you to train them. That's fine – don't push the subject. Keep saying hello and be available if they have questions. When they bring a friend into the gym, take the opportunity to chat with the friend. The more people in the club you know, the better. You'll quickly become the go-to trainer at that club.

This book was brought to you by http://myfitnessentrepreneur.com

About the Author – Ahmed "Gino" Erguigue

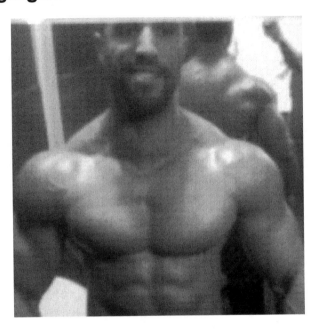

My story

I grew up in Morocco. I always skipped class to play sports and was always getting in trouble. Teachers wanted me to study but all I wanted to do was be outside running track, doing gymnastics, and playing soccer. Basically doing what I love!

Eventually I went to a school for athletics running track and was part of the track and field team. We traveled all over Morocco doing the 100 m, 200 m, and 400 m races (my best time for the 100 m sprint was 10.01 seconds). I loved being involved in sports and it was a big part of my life.

But there was still something missing. I never really felt like I belonged in Morocco. Since I was a kid, I always thought that there were bigger and better things out there for me. I dreamed of Hollywood and the bright and fancy cars and all that you see on television. I was determined to fulfill my dream. I applied to go to the US in customs and I won the lottery! I was given the opportunity to become naturalized as a US citizen. So I packed up my belongings and kissed my family goodbye and moved to the US by myself with nothing but about $300 and not a word of English. Of all the places I could come to in the US, I started out in New York City. I was so scared when I first arrived I even cried. Now 17 years later, and after so much hard work and sacrifice, I am living my dream and doing what I love to do with passion and energy. A career in personal training has made all my dreams come true.

About me

I received my education and training from the **Athletic University of Rabat** (http://www.um5a.ac.ma/index.php/en/), Morocco (the National Academy of Sports Medicine), as well as an extensive amount of practical knowledge gained as a professional track and field athlete. More important than my knowledge of fitness and athleticism is my passion for helping others achieve success in the most important (yet overlooked) aspect of their lives: health and wellness.

The holistic integration of medical knowledge and physical fitness is a combination that is far too often overlooked. My mission is based on the concept of simplifying and building a strong foundation of principles and tools to allow people to live a realistic balanced lifestyle. I am committed to developing customized programs, paralleled with ongoing motivation, that will allow clients to reach their ultimate fitness goals. Changing our bodies is very challenging (just like changing our lifestyle), but with a well defined plan of action to follow, it becomes much more manageable.

My philosophy is based on the concept that we are all on our own journey. Throughout that journey we are continuously learning lessons we need in order to become the most amazing versions of ourselves. With each challenge, we have one choice: to run away or to embrace it and grow as an individual.

Thank you for purchasing and good luck!

Working as a personal trainer for the past 15 years has given me an extremely blessed life and I'm thankful every day that this is my profession. I love the fact that I get paid to positively impact the lives of my clients every single day. I put together this book to to help others achieve a career as rewarding as the one I've experienced. Hopefully this guide will help you find the same joy, satisfaction, and success that I have found in this dynamic profession.

This is my story and I hope you liked it. It came from my heart.

Gino

P.S. – If you have any questions or suggestions on how I can improve this guide, please let me know by contacting me through the contact page of my website! If you like this guide, please share it with anyone who may get some use out of it. That is the best kind of thank you I can get. The other best thank you is to leave a 4 or 5 star review for it on Amazon.

Note: Because recommended equipment and recommended supplements are constantly changing, that information can be found on these pages:

http://myfitnessentrepreneur.com/recommended-equipment/

http://myfitnessentrepreneur.com/recommended-supplements/

Made in the USA
San Bernardino, CA
18 March 2017